Defying the Unseen: Unraveling

Antimicrobial resistance

By

Muhammad Edogi

Table of Contents

Introduction

In the bustling heart of a city, where towering skyscrapers touched the clouds and technology hummed with life, lived a young scientist named Maya. Maya was no ordinary scientist; she had an insatiable curiosity and an unrelenting passion for unraveling the mysteries of the microbial world. Her laboratory was a haven of test tubes, microscopes, and the hum of futuristic machines that seemed to dance to her command.

One day, as Maya peered through her microscope, she stumbled upon a peculiar discovery. In a petri dish filled with harmless bacteria, she noticed a few tiny rebels – microorganisms that defied the antibiotics she had carefully applied. Maya's eyes widened with intrigue, and she knew she had stumbled upon something extraordinary: antimicrobial resistance.

Driven by a fierce determination to understand this newfound phenomenon, Maya dove headfirst into her research. Days turned into nights as she tirelessly delved into the complex interactions between bacteria and antibiotics. Her breakthroughs were nothing short of remarkable; she uncovered the genetic mutations that allowed these microbes to fend off the very medicines designed to defeat them.

But Maya's excitement was tempered by a growing concern. She realized that if left unchecked, antimicrobial resistance could unleash a wave of infections that modern medicine might struggle to control. She couldn't bear the thought of a world where antibiotics, the pillars of medical progress, became ineffective.

Armed with knowledge and a sense of responsibility, Maya embarked on a mission to raise awareness about antimicrobial resistance. She spoke at conferences, engaged with healthcare professionals, and even caught the attention of policymakers. Maya's passion was infectious, and soon, a global movement to combat antimicrobial resistance began to take shape.

As the movement gained momentum, Maya's laboratory became a hub of innovation. Collaborative teams from around the world flocked to her doorstep, eager to join the fight against AMR. Together, they developed new diagnostics that could identify resistant strains within hours, rather than days. They engineered antimicrobial agents that targeted the most stubborn microbes, leaving no room for resistance to take root. And most importantly, they championed the responsible use of antibiotics in healthcare settings, communities, and agriculture.

Maya's story spread far and wide, inspiring individuals to take action in their own spheres. Farmers adopted sustainable practices to prevent the overuse of antibiotics in livestock. Healthcare providers embraced antimicrobial stewardship programs that ensured patients received the right treatment at the right time. Communities rallied together to raise awareness and combat the spread of infections.

Over time, the tide began to turn. Hospitals saw a decline in drug-resistant infections, and lives were saved that would have once been lost to untreatable illnesses. Maya's dedication had ignited a spark that illuminated the path to a future where antibiotics remained effective and humanity triumphed over the formidable threat of antimicrobial resistance.

In the end, Maya's story was not just about scientific discovery; it was a testament to the power of one individual's unwavering passion to catalyze change. And as the city's skyscrapers continued to touch the clouds, Maya's legacy soared even higher – a beacon of hope in a world that had learned to stand united against a microscopic adversary.

Antimicrobial resistance (AMR) refers to the ability of microorganisms, such as bacteria, viruses, fungi, and parasites, to evolve and become resistant to the drugs (antimicrobial agents) that were originally effective in treating infections caused by them. This resistance can render previously treatable infections more difficult to manage and can lead to increased illness, longer recovery times, and even death.

AMR is a serious global public health concern because it threatens the effectiveness of many commonly used antibiotics, antiviral drugs, and other antimicrobial treatments. The misuse and overuse of antimicrobial agents in humans, animals, and agriculture contribute to the development and spread of AMR.

Key points about antimicrobial resistance include:
Causes: AMR arises primarily due to the natural ability of microorganisms to adapt and mutate over time. However, human activities such as inappropriate and excessive use of antibiotics, incomplete treatment regimens, and poor infection control practices accelerate the development and spread of AMR.

1. **Consequences:** As microorganisms become resistant to antimicrobial agents, infections become harder to treat, leading to prolonged illnesses, increased healthcare costs, and higher mortality rates. Procedures such as surgeries, organ transplants, and cancer treatments that rely on effective antimicrobial therapies could become riskier.

2. **One Health Approach:** AMR is not limited to human health; it also affects animals and the environment. The One Health approach recognizes the interconnectedness of human, animal, and environmental health and emphasizes collaborative efforts to combat AMR.

3. **Global Action:** International organizations, governments, healthcare professionals, researchers, and industries are working together to address AMR through strategies such as promoting appropriate antibiotic use, strengthening infection prevention and control measures, and investing in research for new antimicrobial drugs.

4. **Diagnostic Development:** Improved diagnostics are crucial to identifying the specific

pathogens causing infections and determining their susceptibility to different antimicrobial agents. This helps healthcare providers prescribe targeted treatments and reduce unnecessary antibiotic use.

5. **New Drug Development:** The discovery and development of new antimicrobial drugs, including antibiotics, antiviral, and antifungal agents, are essential to combating AMR. However, the development of new drugs is challenging and often faces scientific, regulatory, and economic hurdles.

6. **Public Awareness:** Raising awareness among the general public, healthcare professionals, and policymakers about the importance of responsible antimicrobial use and the risks associated with AMR is a critical step in tackling the issue.

In summary, antimicrobial resistance poses a significant threat to public health and necessitates a comprehensive and coordinated global effort to ensure the continued effectiveness of antimicrobial treatments. Addressing AMR requires collaboration between healthcare sectors, governments, industries, and individuals to promote responsible antimicrobial use, develop new treatment options, and implement effective infection prevention and control measures.

Antimicrobial Resistance: Understanding its Mechanisms, Causes, and Implications

Antimicrobial resistance (AMR) is a pressing global health challenge that threatens the effectiveness of essential medications used to treat infections caused by bacteria, viruses, fungi, and parasites. The evolution of AMR is a complex process driven by various genetic, ecological, and behavioral factors. This essay delves into the mechanisms, causes, and implications of antimicrobial resistance, shedding light on the multifaceted nature of this issue.

Mechanisms of Antimicrobial Resistance:

AMR develops through several interconnected mechanisms that enable microorganisms to withstand the effects of antimicrobial agents. These mechanisms can be broadly categorized into the following:

1. **Genetic Mutation:** Microorganisms possess the inherent ability to mutate and acquire genetic changes over time. Mutations can lead to alterations in the targets of antimicrobial drugs,

rendering them less effective. For instance, bacteria can modify the structure of their cell walls or enzymes targeted by antibiotics, thereby reducing drug binding and neutralizing their effects.

2. **Horizontal Gene Transfer:** Microorganisms can transfer resistance genes horizontally between different species, promoting the rapid spread of resistance traits. This can occur through mechanisms such as conjugation, transformation, and transduction. The transfer of resistance genes contributes to the emergence of multidrug-resistant strains.

3. **Efflux Pumps:** Some microorganisms develop efflux pumps, specialized proteins that actively pump out antimicrobial agents from within the cell before they can exert their effects. This mechanism allows microorganisms to maintain low intracellular drug concentrations, reducing the drug's efficacy.

4. **Biofuel Formation:** Biofilms are complex communities of microorganisms encased in a protective matrix. Within biofilms, microorganisms are more resistant to antimicrobial agents due to physical barriers

and altered metabolic states. This phenomenon is particularly relevant in chronic infections and medical device-associated infections.

Causes of Antimicrobial Resistance:

AMR is a result of the interplay between biological, environmental, and societal factors. Several key causes contribute to the development and spread of antimicrobial resistance:

1. **Inappropriate Antibiotic Use:** The misuse and overuse of antibiotics in human and veterinary medicine provide selection pressure for resistant strains to emerge. Factors such as unnecessary prescriptions, improper dosing, and patient noncompliance contribute to this issue.

2. **Suboptimal Infection Control:** Poor infection prevention and control practices in healthcare settings can facilitate the transmission of drug-resistant pathogens. Inadequate sanitation, insufficient hand hygiene, and contaminated medical equipment contribute to the spread of AMR.

3. **Antibiotic Use in Agriculture:** The use of antibiotics in livestock and agriculture for

growth promotion and disease prevention can lead to the emergence of resistant bacteria. Resistant bacteria from animals can enter the food chain and impact human health.

4. **Global Travel and Trade:** International travel and trade facilitate the rapid dissemination of resistant microorganisms across borders. Resistant strains can be carried by individuals, animals, or contaminated goods, contributing to the global spread of AMR.

5. **Lack of New Drug Development:** The pipeline for new antimicrobial drug development has significantly diminished over the years due to scientific, regulatory, and economic challenges. The absence of effective treatment options exacerbates the AMR crisis.

6. **Environmental Factors:** Environmental contamination with antimicrobial residues from pharmaceutical manufacturing, agriculture, and healthcare settings can contribute to the selection and spread of resistant strains in the environment.

The consequences of AMR are far-reaching and affect various aspects of healthcare, society, and the economy:

1. **Increased Morbidity and Mortality**: Resistant infections are often more difficult to treat, leading to longer illness durations, increased hospitalizations, and higher mortality rates. Routine medical procedures, such as surgeries and chemotherapy, become riskier.

2. **Healthcare Costs**: The management of AMR-related infections is associated with higher healthcare costs due to prolonged hospital stays, increased use of expensive drugs, and the need for specialized care.

3. **Economic Impact**: AMR can impact economies by reducing workforce productivity, increasing treatment expenses, and straining healthcare systems.

4. **Loss of Medical Advances**: Without effective antimicrobial agents, medical advancements such as organ transplants, cancer treatments, and complex surgeries may become more challenging or even untenable.

5. **One Health Impact**: AMR affects not only human health but also animal health and the environment. The interconnectedness of these domains underscores the importance of a One Health approach to combating AMR.
6. **Global Health Security**: AMR poses a threat to global health security, as it can undermine our ability to respond effectively to infectious disease outbreaks and pandemics.

Antimicrobial resistance is a multifaceted phenomenon driven by intricate genetic mechanisms and influenced by a range of interconnected causes. The development and spread of resistance jeopardize the efficacy of essential antimicrobial agents and have far-reaching implications for healthcare, society, and the global economy. Addressing AMR requires a collaborative effort involving healthcare professionals, policymakers, researchers, and the public to implement effective strategies for responsible antimicrobial use, infection prevention, and new drug development. Only through comprehensive and concerted action can we hope to mitigate the impact of antimicrobial resistance and ensure the continued effectiveness of antimicrobial therapies.

Certainly, here are five important things to know about antimicrobial resistance:

Definition and Scope:

Antimicrobial resistance (AMR) refers to the ability of microorganisms, such as bacteria, viruses, fungi, and parasites, to evolve and develop resistance to the drugs (antimicrobial agents) that were originally effective in treating infections. It is a global health concern that affects human, animal, and environmental health.

Causes and Contributing Factors:

AMR arises primarily from the misuse and overuse of antimicrobial agents. Factors such as inappropriate antibiotic prescribing, patient noncompliance with treatment regimens, use of antibiotics in livestock and agriculture, poor infection control practices, and lack of new drug development all contribute to the development and spread of AMR.

Impact on Health and Healthcare:

AMR has significant implications for public health. Resistant infections are more difficult to treat, leading to longer hospital stays, increased healthcare costs, and higher mortality rates. Routine medical procedures, from surgeries to cancer treatments, become riskier due to the potential for treatment failure.

Addressing AMR requires a coordinated effort across sectors and countries. The One Health approach recognizes the interconnectedness of human health, animal health, and the environment. It emphasizes the need for collaboration between healthcare, veterinary, and environmental sectors to combat AMR effectively.

Prevention and Mitigation Strategies:

Several strategies are crucial in tackling AMR:

Responsible Antibiotic Use: Healthcare professionals should prescribe antibiotics judiciously, following guidelines and considering the appropriate drug, dose, and duration.

- Infection Prevention and Control: Proper hygiene practices, sanitation, and infection control measures in healthcare settings help reduce the spread of resistant pathogens.
- Vaccination: Immunization can prevent some infections, reducing the need for antimicrobial treatment.

- ➤ Public Awareness: Raising awareness among the public, healthcare providers, and policymakers about the risks of AMR and the importance of responsible antimicrobial use is essential.
- ➤ Research and Innovation: Investment in research for new antimicrobial agents, diagnostics, and treatment alternatives is critical to address the evolving challenge of AMR.

Understanding these key aspects of antimicrobial resistance is crucial for individuals, healthcare systems, and societies to take effective actions to combat this growing threat to global health.

COVID-19 & Antimicrobial Resistance

COVID-19 and antimicrobial resistance (AMR) are two distinct global health challenges, but they share certain similarities and interactions that have important implications for public health. Here's an overview of the relationship between COVID-19 and AMR:

1. Distinct Challenges:

COVID-19: COVID-19 is a viral respiratory illness caused by the severe acute respiratory syndrome corona virus 2 (SARS-CoV-2). It primarily affects the respiratory system and has led to a global pandemic, with significant morbidity and mortality.

Antimicrobial Resistance: AMR involves the ability of microorganisms (e.g., bacteria, viruses, fungi) to develop resistance to drugs, particularly antibiotics and antiviral. This resistance can render infections more difficult to treat and can lead to increased illness and death.

2. Interactions and Overlapping Concerns:

Antibiotics and COVID-19: During the COVID-19 pandemic, there has been concern about the overuse and inappropriate use of antibiotics in patients with viral infections like COVID-19. This misuse contributes to the development of antibiotic resistance.

Secondary Infections: COVID-19 patients are at risk of developing secondary bacterial infections, which may lead to increased antibiotic use. AMR could exacerbate these infections, making treatment more challenging.

3. Impact on Healthcare Systems:

Strain on Healthcare Resources: Both COVID-19 and AMR can strain healthcare systems. An increased demand for medical care due to COVID-19 can divert resources from addressing AMR, and vice versa.

Risk of Co-Infections: Patients with severe COVID-19 are vulnerable to bacterial co-infections, which may require antibiotics. This further highlights the need for judicious antibiotic use to prevent AMR.

4. One Health Approach: Shared Environment: Both COVID-19 and AMR emphasize the importance of a One Health approach, recognizing the interconnectedness of human, animal, and environmental health. The misuse of antibiotics in animal agriculture can contribute to AMR, while zoonotic diseases like COVID-19 highlight the link between animal and human health.

5. Public Health Response:

Prevention Strategies: Public health measures to control COVID-19 (e.g., vaccination, infection control) also align with strategies to prevent AMR (e.g., responsible antibiotic use, infection prevention).

Research and Innovation: The urgency to develop vaccines and treatments for COVID-19 has underscored the importance of research and innovation. A similar approach is needed to develop new antimicrobial agents to combat AMR.

6. Lessons and Moving Forward:

Behavioral Change: The global response to COVID-19 has shown that behavioral change (e.g., hand hygiene, mask-wearing) can be effective in controlling infectious diseases. Similar efforts are needed to address AMR through responsible antimicrobial use.

Global Collaboration: The international collaboration seen during the COVID-19 pandemic can serve as a model for addressing AMR. Multilateral efforts are essential to combat both challenges effectively.

while COVID-19 and antimicrobial resistance are distinct challenges, their interactions and shared concerns highlight the importance of responsible antimicrobial use, infection prevention, and global cooperation. As we continue to address the COVID-19 pandemic, it is imperative that we also prioritize efforts to mitigate the development and spread of antimicrobial resistance to safeguard public health for the long term.

Microbial ecology is a branch of ecology that focuses on the interactions, relationships, and dynamics of microorganisms within various environments. Microorganisms, including bacteria, archaea, viruses, fungi, and protists, play fundamental roles in ecosystems, affecting nutrient cycling, energy flow, and overall ecosystem health. Microbial ecology studies the diversity, distribution, abundance, and activities of these microorganisms and how they interact with each other and their surroundings.

Key Concepts in Microbial Ecology:

➢ Microbial Diversity: Microbial ecosystems are incredibly diverse and can be found in almost every imaginable habitat, including soil, water bodies, sediments, plants, animals, and extreme environments like hot springs and deep-sea hydrothermal vents. Microbial diversity refers to the variety of different microorganisms present in these habitats.

➢ Microbial Interactions: Microorganisms interact with each other and with their environment in complex ways. These interactions include competition for resources, mutualism (beneficial interactions), predation, parasitism, and symbiosis.

➢ Nutrient Cycling: Microorganisms are critical in nutrient cycling processes, such as nitrogen fixation, gentrification, carbon cycling, and sulfur cycling. They break down organic matter, release nutrients, and transform compounds into forms usable by other organisms.

➢ Biogeochemical Cycling: Microbial activity directly impacts the movement of elements (e.g., carbon, nitrogen, phosphorus) between the living and non-living components of ecosystems. Biogeochemical cycles involve the cycling of elements through various microbial processes.

➢ Community Structure: Microbial communities are composed of different species with varying roles and functions. Studying community structure involves understanding how these species coexist, compete, and contribute to ecosystem functioning.

➢ Ecological Niches: Microorganisms occupy specific ecological niches within ecosystems based on factors like temperature, pH, availability of nutrients, and interactions with other organisms. These niches shape the distribution and abundance of different microbial populations.

➤ Ecosystem Health and Resilience: Microbial communities play a crucial role in maintaining ecosystem health and resilience. Changes in microbial populations can impact nutrient availability, disease dynamics, and overall ecosystem stability.

➤ Micro biomes: A microbiome refers to the collection of microorganisms, their genomes, and their environmental interactions within a particular habitat or organism. The human gut microbiome, for example, has been extensively studied for its influence on human health.

➤ Emergent Properties: Microbial ecosystems exhibit emergent properties, where the interactions among microorganisms give rise to system-level behaviors that cannot be predicted from studying individual microorganisms alone.

➤ Applied Microbial Ecology: Microbial ecology has practical applications in various fields, such as agriculture, bioremediation (using microorganisms to clean up pollutants), wastewater treatment, disease control, and biotechnology.

Overall, microbial ecology provides insights into the intricate relationships and processes that shape ecosystems and influence the functioning of our planet. Studying microbial communities and their interactions enhances our understanding of how ecosystems work, how they respond to disturbances, and how they can be managed sustainably.

Where Resistance Spreads: Exploring the Pathways of Antimicrobial Resistance Dissemination

Antimicrobial resistance (AMR) is a complex and multifaceted global challenge that impacts various aspects of public health, environmental ecosystems, and global trade. The spread of resistance occurs through interconnected pathways that traverse healthcare facilities, local communities, water and soil environments, the food supply chain, and across international borders. Understanding these pathways is crucial for devising effective strategies to mitigate the spread of AMR and preserve the efficacy of antimicrobial agents.

Healthcare Facilities:

Healthcare settings play a pivotal role in the emergence and dissemination of antimicrobial resistance. Hospitals, clinics, and other medical institutions provide environments where both susceptible and resistant microorganisms coexist. Factors contributing to the spread of resistance in healthcare facilities include:

- Overuse of Antibiotics: Excessive and inappropriate use of antibiotics in healthcare settings can lead to the development of resistant strains. Broad-spectrum antibiotics are often prescribed when they are not necessary, promoting the growth of resistant bacteria.
- Hospital Acquired Infections: Resistant infections acquired during hospital stays, often referred to as healthcare-associated infections (HAIs) or nosocomial infections, pose a significant risk to patients. The close proximity of patients, invasive medical procedures, and prolonged antibiotic use contribute to the spread of resistant strains.
- Lack of Infection Control: Inadequate hygiene practices, poor sanitation, and inadequate infection control measures can facilitate the transmission of resistant microorganisms within healthcare facilities.
- Horizontal Gene Transfer: The exchange of resistance genes between different bacteria can occur within healthcare environments, leading to the rapid dissemination of resistance traits.

The spread of AMR extends beyond healthcare facilities and into local communities, where factors such as personal behaviors, public health measures, and socioeconomic conditions can influence resistance dissemination:

> ➤ Over-the-Counter Antibiotics: Access to over-the-counter antibiotics in some countries allows individuals to self-medicate, often leading to inappropriate and inadequate use of antibiotics, which contributes to resistance development.

> ➤ Incomplete Treatment: Failure to complete a prescribed course of antibiotics can result in the survival of partially resistant microorganisms, potentially leading to the emergence of more resistant strains.

> ➤ Livestock and Agriculture: The use of antibiotics in agriculture can introduce resistant bacteria into the environment, impacting local ecosystems and potentially affecting human health through the food chain.

> ➤ Poor Sanitation: Inadequate sanitation and wastewater management can lead to the release of antimicrobial agents and resistant bacteria

into the environment, contaminating water sources and soil.

Water & Soil:

The environment, particularly water bodies and soil, serves as a reservoir for antimicrobial resistance. Several factors contribute to the spread of resistance in these ecosystems:

> Antibiotic Residues: The release of antibiotics and their metabolites into water bodies, often from agricultural runoff and pharmaceutical manufacturing, can exert selective pressure on microorganisms and promote resistance.

> Wastewater Discharge: Wastewater from hospitals and households can carry resistant bacteria and antibiotic residues into water bodies. Resistant bacteria present in water can be transmitted to humans through recreational activities or consumption of contaminated water or seafood.

> Biofilm Formation: Microorganisms in aquatic environments can form biofilms, protective structures that facilitate the exchange of genetic material, including resistance genes.

➢ Soil as Reservoir: Soil can serve as a reservoir for resistant microorganisms due to the widespread use of antibiotics in agriculture. Resistance genes can also transfer between soil bacteria.

The food supply chain is another crucial pathway for the dissemination of AMR. Resistant microorganisms can be transmitted to humans through consumption of contaminated food:

➢ Animal Farming: The use of antibiotics in animal agriculture for growth promotion and disease prevention can lead to the development of resistant strains in animals. These strains can then be transmitted to humans through consumption of meat, poultry, and dairy products.

➢ Aquaculture: The use of antibiotics in aquaculture can promote resistance in fish and seafood, which can subsequently be transmitted to humans.

➢ Food Processing: Cross-contamination of resistant bacteria during food processing can lead to the presence of resistant microorganisms in ready-to-eat products.

- ➤ International Trade: The global movement of food products can facilitate the spread of resistant microorganisms across borders, contributing to the global dissemination of AMR.

Antimicrobial resistance is a global concern that transcends national boundaries and requires international collaboration to address effectively:

- ➤ International Travel: People traveling across countries can carry resistant microorganisms with them, potentially contributing to the spread of resistance globally.
- ➤ Medical Tourism: Medical procedures conducted abroad, particularly in regions with less stringent infection control measures, can expose patients to resistant microorganisms.
- ➤ Trade and Migration: The movement of goods and people across borders can facilitate the transmission of resistant strains and resistance genes between different regions.
- ➤ Global Health Security: AMR poses a threat to global health security by reducing the effectiveness of treatments for infectious

diseases, including those with pandemic potential, such as COVID-19.

The spread of antimicrobial resistance occurs through a complex web of pathways that encompass healthcare facilities, local communities, water and soil environments, the food supply chain, and international interactions. Addressing this challenge requires a multifaceted approach that involves responsible antibiotic use, improved infection control, proper waste management, sustainable agricultural practices, and international cooperation. By understanding and targeting the various pathways of resistance dissemination, we can work toward preserving the effectiveness of antimicrobial agents and safeguarding human and environmental health on a global scale.

Actions to Fight Antimicrobial Resistance: Strategies for Mitigating the Global Health Crisis

Antimicrobial resistance (AMR) poses a significant threat to human and animal health, as well as to the environment. Addressing this complex challenge requires coordinated efforts at various levels, from individual actions to policy interventions. The following sections delve into strategies and actions that can be taken by individuals, healthcare providers, health departments, veterinarian practices, and livestock and poultry producers to combat AMR.

Protect Yourself and Your Family:

1. Responsible Antibiotic Use: Follow healthcare professionals' advice when prescribed antibiotics. Always complete the full course of antibiotics even if you start feeling better, as incomplete treatment can promote the emergence of resistant bacteria.

2. Vaccination: Stay up-to-date with vaccinations to prevent infections that might lead to unnecessary antibiotic use.

3. Hand Hygiene: Regularly wash your hands with soap and water to reduce the risk of infections and the need for antibiotics.
4. Infection Prevention: Practice good hygiene, such as covering your mouth when you cough or sneeze, to prevent the spread of infections.
5. Food Safety: Handle and prepare food properly to avoid food borne illnesses that might necessitate antibiotic treatment.
6. Avoid Antibiotics for Viral Infections: Antibiotics are ineffective against viral infections like colds, flu, and most sore throats. Using antibiotics for such infections can contribute to antibiotic resistance.
7. Limit Over-the-Counter Use: Avoid using over-the-counter antibiotics without a prescription, as improper use can lead to resistance.

Healthcare Providers:

➢ Prescribe Appropriately: Only prescribe antibiotics when they are truly needed. Follow evidence-based guidelines to choose the right antibiotic, dose, and duration.
➢ Implement Stewardship Programs: Establish antimicrobial stewardship programs in healthcare facilities to promote appropriate

antibiotic use, monitor resistance patterns, and improve patient outcomes.

> Rapid Diagnostics: Use rapid diagnostic tests to identify the specific pathogens causing infections, allowing targeted antibiotic treatment.

> Patient Education: Educate patients about the proper use of antibiotics, the importance of completing treatment, and the consequences of resistance.

> Infection Control: Implement robust infection control measures in healthcare settings to prevent the spread of resistant pathogens among patients and healthcare workers.

Health Departments:

> Surveillance and Monitoring: Establish systems to monitor the prevalence of antimicrobial resistance in different healthcare settings and the community.

> Education and Awareness: Launch public awareness campaigns to educate the public, healthcare providers, and veterinarians about the risks of AMR and the importance of responsible antimicrobial use.

- ➤ Regulation and Policy: Develop and enforce regulations to ensure the proper use of antibiotics in healthcare and agriculture, as well as proper waste disposal to prevent environmental contamination.
- ➤ Collaboration: Facilitate collaboration between healthcare, agriculture, environmental, and research sectors to implement a One Health approach to address AMR.

Veterinarian Practices:

1. Judicious Use of Antibiotics: Veterinarians should prescribe antibiotics only when necessary for animal health and welfare. Consider alternatives such as vaccines and improved management practices.
2. Veterinary Oversight: Establish veterinary-client-patient relationships to ensure responsible use of antibiotics in animals. Regularly review and update treatment protocols.
3. Preventive Measures: Emphasize preventive measures, such as proper hygiene, biosecurity, and vaccination, to reduce the need for antibiotics.

4. Responsible Drug Selection: Choose antibiotics that are effective for specific bacterial infections and minimize the use of medically important antibiotics in animals that are crucial for human health.

➤ Reduce Antibiotic Use: Adopt practices that minimize the need for antibiotics in animal production, such as improving hygiene, nutrition, and animal housing conditions.

➤ Veterinary Guidance: Work closely with veterinarians to develop herd health management plans that prioritize animal health while minimizing the use of antibiotics.

➤ Selective Breeding: Focus on breeding animals that are more resilient to diseases, reducing the need for antibiotics.

➤ Antibiotic Alternatives: Invest in research and development of alternatives to antibiotics, such as probiotics, probiotics, and innovative feed additives.

➤ Record Keeping: Maintain accurate records of antibiotic use and animal health outcomes, allowing for informed decision-making and transparency.

➢ Fighting antimicrobial resistance requires a comprehensive and collaborative effort that spans individual actions, healthcare settings, regulatory bodies, veterinary practices, and agricultural sectors. By implementing responsible antibiotic use, improving infection control measures, and promoting awareness, we can work together to slow the emergence and spread of AMR. Recognizing the interconnectedness of human, animal, and environmental health, a One Health approach is essential to effectively combat this global health crisis.

What CDC Is Doing: Investments & U.S. Action in the Fight against Antimicrobial Resistance

The Centers for Disease Control and Prevention (CDC) plays a pivotal role in addressing the global challenge of antimicrobial resistance (AMR). Through strategic investments and coordinated efforts, the CDC is at the forefront of combating AMR in the United States and around the world. This section delves into the multifaceted approach adopted by the CDC, including its investment initiatives, collaborative actions, and innovative strategies to tackle AMR.

Investment Map: Funding in Your State

The CDC's commitment to addressing AMR is evident through its comprehensive funding initiatives aimed at supporting AMR research, surveillance, and prevention efforts across all states in the U.S. The CDC's investment map provides a transparent view of the funding allocations to each state, illustrating the agency's dedication to a nationwide approach in the fight against AMR. By channeling resources into state-level activities, the CDC is empowering local communities, healthcare facilities, and public health departments to actively engage in AMR prevention and control.

Healthcare Action: Enhancing Antimicrobial Stewardship

One of the CDC's key focuses is on healthcare settings, where the agency promotes the responsible use of antibiotics through antimicrobial stewardship programs. These programs emphasize the appropriate prescribing and use of antibiotics, ensuring that patients receive the right antibiotic, at the right dose, and for the right duration. The CDC's efforts include providing guidelines, tools, and resources to healthcare providers, hospitals, and clinics, enabling them to implement effective stewardship measures that combat AMR while optimizing patient care.

Community Action: Engaging Local Communities

Recognizing the importance of community engagement, the CDC works to raise awareness about AMR and empower individuals to take action. Through educational campaigns, the CDC educates the public about the risks of AMR, the role of responsible antibiotic use, and preventive measures to reduce the spread of infections. By fostering a sense of collective responsibility, the CDC encourages communities to contribute to the fight against AMR.

Environment Action: Addressing Environmental Factors

The CDC recognizes the critical role of the environment in the spread of AMR. The agency collaborates with partners to assess the impact of antimicrobial use in agriculture, pharmaceutical manufacturing, and healthcare on environmental AMR. By studying environmental factors, the CDC aims to better understand the pathways of resistance dissemination and develop strategies to mitigate environmental contributions to AMR.

Food Supply Action: Safeguarding the Food Chain

Ensuring the safety of the food supply is a paramount concern for the CDC. The agency collaborates with the U.S. Department of Agriculture (USDA) and the Food and Drug Administration (FDA) to monitor and address AMR in the food chain. By conducting surveillance of resistant pathogens in food and animals, the CDC informs policies and interventions that promote responsible antibiotic use in agriculture and minimize the transmission of resistant bacteria to humans through food consumption.

The CDC's commitment to global health is evident through its efforts to combat AMR on a global scale. The agency collaborates with international partners, including the World Health Organization (WHO) and other nations, to develop strategies for AMR surveillance, prevention, and control. Through capacity-building initiatives and knowledge-sharing, the CDC contributes to a collective effort to address the transnational challenge of AMR.

Rapid and accurate diagnostics are vital in the fight against AMR. The CDC supports laboratories across the U.S. in enhancing their capacity to detect and characterize resistant microorganisms. By providing training, technical assistance, and state-of-the-art tools, the CDC empowers laboratories to identify and monitor AMR effectively, enabling timely and informed clinical decision-making.

Innovation is a cornerstone of the CDC's approach to tackling AMR. The agency conducts groundbreaking research to advance our understanding of AMR mechanisms, transmission dynamics, and prevention strategies. By fostering innovation in diagnostics, treatment, and infection control, the CDC contributes to the development of novel solutions to combat AMR and protect public health.

U.S. Action & Events: Mobilizing National Efforts

The CDC's AMR activities extend to mobilizing national initiatives and events that highlight the importance of addressing AMR. Through observances like Antibiotic Awareness Week, the CDC raises awareness about the urgent need for responsible antibiotic use and the consequences of AMR. By engaging healthcare professionals, policymakers, and the public, the CDC amplifies its efforts to drive meaningful change.

Apply for CDC Funding: Empowering Local Solutions

Recognizing the significance of grassroots efforts, the CDC provides opportunities for organizations and communities to access funding for AMR-related projects. By offering grants and cooperative agreements, the CDC empowers stakeholders to implement innovative interventions, research studies, and educational campaigns that contribute to the fight against AMR. Through these funding mechanisms, the CDC fosters diverse and impactful initiatives that collectively contribute to AMR prevention and control.

The CDC's multifaceted approach to addressing antimicrobial resistance encompasses strategic investments, collaborative actions, and innovative strategies. From healthcare facilities and local communities to global partnerships and research endeavors, the CDC's efforts span a spectrum of activities that collectively aim to mitigate the threat of AMR. By championing responsible antibiotic use, strengthening diagnostics, and fostering innovation, the CDC plays a pivotal role in safeguarding public health and ensuring the efficacy of antimicrobial agents for generations to come.

National Infection & Death Estimates: Unveiling the Burden of Antimicrobial Resistance

Antimicrobial resistance (AMR) is a global health crisis that exacts a significant toll on human health and healthcare systems. National infection and death estimates provide critical insights into the scale of this challenge, enabling policymakers, healthcare professionals, and the public to grasp the magnitude of AMR's impact. This section explores the importance of national infection and death estimates in shedding light on the burden of AMR and guiding effective interventions.

AMR-associated infections result in substantial morbidity and mortality, straining healthcare resources and challenging medical treatment. National infection estimates quantify the number of infections caused by resistant microorganisms, encompassing a wide spectrum of pathogens such as bacteria, viruses, fungi, and parasites. These estimates take into account healthcare-associated infections (HAIs), community-acquired infections, and infections acquired through various routes.

National death estimates, on the other hand, reveal the human toll of AMR by quantifying the number of deaths attributed to resistant infections. These estimates underscore the urgent need to address AMR as a public health priority, motivating actions that aim to reduce the impact of resistant infections on individuals and communities.

The collection and analysis of data for national infection and death estimates involve robust surveillance systems, laboratory diagnostics, and collaboration between healthcare institutions, public health agencies, and researchers. By combining clinical data, epidemiological investigations, and advanced modeling techniques, these estimates provide a comprehensive overview of the burden of AMR at the national level.

The dissemination of national infection and death estimates is a vital step in raising awareness and advocating for policy changes. These estimates inform healthcare guidelines, resource allocation, and interventions to prevent and control AMR. Additionally, they enable comparisons between different regions, highlighting variations in AMR burden and aiding in the identification of high-risk populations or geographic areas.

National infection and death estimates serve as powerful tools in revealing the true extent of the AMR crisis. By quantifying the infections and deaths attributed to resistant microorganisms, these estimates drive the formulation of evidence-based strategies to combat AMR, improve patient outcomes, and ensure the sustainability of antimicrobial therapies.

AR Threats Report: Unveiling the Landscape of Antimicrobial Resistance Threats

The Antimicrobial Resistance (AR) Threats Report is a cornerstone publication that illuminates the evolving landscape of AMR, providing a comprehensive assessment of the current state of antimicrobial resistance and its implications for public health. This report, compiled by health agencies such as the Centers for Disease Control and Prevention (CDC), underscores the urgency of addressing AMR and informs strategies to mitigate its impact.

The AR Threats Report categorizes pathogens into three tiers: urgent, serious, and concerning. These classifications reflect the level of threat posed by resistant microorganisms based on factors such as clinical impact, prevalence, and available treatment options. The report also highlights specific pathogens and infections, including drug-resistant tuberculosis, carbapenem-resistant Enterobacterales, and Clostridioides difficile infections, shedding light on emerging and reemerging challenges.

In addition to pathogen-specific assessments, the AR Threats Report examines the broader consequences of AMR, encompassing healthcare-associated infections, community-acquired infections, and infections acquired through various routes. The report underscores the economic burden of AMR, the challenges of antimicrobial development, and the potential for AMR to undermine medical advances and public health achievements.

The AR Threats Report emphasizes the interconnectedness of human health, animal health, and the environment in the spread of AMR. It underscores the importance of a One Health approach that recognizes the shared responsibility of various sectors in combatting AMR.

Publications, such as the AR Threats Report, play a crucial role in guiding policy decisions, shaping healthcare guidelines, and driving public awareness campaigns. By presenting a comprehensive overview of AMR threats, these reports empower governments, healthcare professionals, researchers, and the public to take informed actions that collectively contribute to the containment of AMR.

The AR Threats Report serves as a beacon of knowledge, illuminating the multifaceted challenges posed by AMR. By providing a clear picture of the current and potential impact of resistant microorganisms, this report catalyzes efforts to address AMR, encourages collaborative approaches, and emphasizes the necessity of a concerted global response.

Tracking Resistance: Surveillance and Data Collection for Informed Action

Surveillance and data collection are essential pillars of the global effort to combat antimicrobial resistance (AMR). These processes involve systematic monitoring of resistant microorganisms, their prevalence, and their patterns of resistance to various antimicrobial agents. By tracking resistance over time, surveillance programs provide crucial insights into the changing dynamics of AMR, enabling informed decision-making, policy formulation, and targeted interventions.

Surveillance efforts encompass a range of settings, including healthcare facilities, communities, agriculture, and the environment. These initiatives involve the collection and analysis of clinical and microbiological data from diverse sources, such as hospitals, laboratories, veterinary practices, and public health agencies. The data collected includes information on the type of microorganisms, the antimicrobial agents to which they are resistant, and patient outcomes.

Several key elements are fundamental to effective surveillance and data collection for AMR:

Standardized Protocols: Establishing consistent and standardized protocols for data collection, laboratory testing, and reporting ensures the accuracy and comparability of surveillance data.

Multidisciplinary Collaboration: Successful surveillance requires collaboration between healthcare professionals, veterinarians, researchers, and public health officials. This multidisciplinary approach facilitates the integration of data from various sectors.

Rapid Diagnostics: The availability of rapid diagnostic tests allows for timely identification of resistant microorganisms, enabling prompt clinical decision-making and appropriate patient management.

Technological Advancements: Advances in sequencing technologies and bioinformatics enhance the ability to track the genetic mechanisms underlying resistance and trace the spread of resistant strains.

International Cooperation: AMR is a global challenge, and international collaboration is essential for harmonizing surveillance efforts, sharing data, and addressing cross-border transmission.

Surveillance data provide a basis for evidence-based interventions to prevent and control AMR. They enable healthcare providers to make informed treatment decisions, guide the development of antimicrobial stewardship programs, and support the implementation of infection prevention and control measures.

Moreover, surveillance data serve as a foundation for policy advocacy and resource allocation. Governments, public health agencies, and international organizations use this data to shape policies, allocate funding, and prioritize interventions aimed at curbing the spread of AMR.

Tracking resistance through robust surveillance and data collection is indispensable in the fight against AMR. By generating insights into resistance patterns, identifying emerging threats, and informing targeted interventions, surveillance programs play a pivotal role in safeguarding the effectiveness of antimicrobial agents and preserving human and animal health.

Publications with Data: Building a Knowledge Base for Informed AMR Interventions

Publications that present data on antimicrobial resistance (AMR) are invaluable resources that contribute to the understanding of the complex dynamics surrounding this global health challenge. These publications provide critical insights into the prevalence, mechanisms, and consequences of AMR, informing evidence-based interventions, guiding policy decisions, and shaping the future direction of AMR control efforts.

These publications encompass a wide range of formats, including research articles, epidemiological reports, surveillance summaries, and reviews. They draw from diverse data sources, such as clinical specimens, microbiological testing, patient outcomes, and genetic analyses of resistant microorganisms.

Key aspects of publications with AMR data include:

> Epidemiological Analysis: Publications often analyze epidemiological data to assess the prevalence of resistant microorganisms, patterns of resistance, and risk factors associated with AMR.

> Mechanisms of Resistance: Data-driven studies delve into the genetic and molecular mechanisms underlying resistance, shedding light on how microorganisms evade the effects of antimicrobial agents.

> Impact and Consequences: Publications explore the clinical, economic, and societal impact of AMR, highlighting the increased morbidity, mortality, and healthcare costs associated with resistant infections.

> Geographic and Temporal Trends: By analyzing data from different regions and over time,

publications reveal geographic variations in AMR prevalence and trends in resistance emergence and spread.

One Health Approach: Many publications adopt a One Health perspective, recognizing the interconnectedness of human health, animal health, and the environment in the dissemination of AMR.

- ➤ Surveillance and Monitoring: Publications often present findings from surveillance programs that track resistance in healthcare facilities, communities, and various sectors.
- ➤ The insights derived from publications with AMR data inform a spectrum of actions:
- ➤ Clinical Decision-Making: Healthcare professionals use data to make informed treatment choices, optimize patient care, and implement antimicrobial stewardship programs.
- ➤ Policy Formulation: Governments and public health agencies utilize data to shape policies, regulations, and interventions aimed at preventing and controlling AMR.
- ➤ Research Prioritization: Researchers identify gaps in knowledge, prioritize research

questions, and develop innovative approaches to combat AMR.

➤ Education and Awareness: Publications contribute to educational initiatives that raise awareness about AMR among healthcare providers, policymakers, and the general public.

➤ Global Collaboration: International organizations use data to facilitate cross-border collaboration, harmonize surveillance efforts, and coordinate strategies to address AMR.

Publications with AMR data play a pivotal role in building a comprehensive knowledge base that informs strategies to combat AMR. By disseminating evidence, driving informed actions, and fostering collaborative efforts, these publications contribute to the global endeavor to mitigate the threat of antimicrobial resistance and preserve the effectiveness of antimicrobial agents.

Communication Resources: Empowering Action Against Antimicrobial Resistance

Effective communication is a cornerstone of efforts to combat antimicrobial resistance (AMR). By disseminating accurate and accessible information, communication resources empower individuals, healthcare professionals, policymakers, and communities to take informed actions to prevent and control AMR. This section explores a range of communication tools, from print materials and fact sheets to digital resources, press releases, and feature stories, that collectively contribute to raising awareness and driving meaningful change in the fight against AMR.

Print Materials & Fact Sheets: Knowledge in Your Hands

Print materials and fact sheets are tangible resources that distill complex information about AMR into accessible formats. These materials provide clear and concise explanations of key concepts related to AMR, including the importance of responsible antibiotic use, infection prevention strategies, and the consequences of AMR for public health.

Key elements of effective print materials and fact sheets include:

> ➢ Clarity and Accessibility: Content is presented in simple language, making it understandable to a broad audience, including individuals with varying levels of health literacy.
> ➢ Visual Aids: Info graphics, illustrations, and charts enhance understanding and retention of information, conveying key messages at a glance.
> ➢ Actionable Tips: Practical recommendations empower readers with actionable steps they can take to prevent AMR, such as practicing good hand hygiene and completing prescribed antibiotic courses.
> ➢ Source Attribution: References and sources lend credibility to the information presented, instilling trust in the accuracy of the content.

Print materials and fact sheets serve as educational tools for healthcare settings, community events, schools, and workplaces. They are valuable resources for empowering individuals with the knowledge and motivation to make informed decisions in their daily lives.

In the digital age, online platforms offer a dynamic and far-reaching means of communication. Digital resources, including social media posts and videos, leverage the power of visual and interactive content to engage audiences and convey messages effectively.

Social Media Campaigns: Platforms like Twitter, Facebook, and Instagram enable organizations like the CDC to launch targeted social media campaigns that amplify key messages about AMR. Campaigns may include hash tags, info graphics, and short videos that raise awareness and drive conversations.

Educational Videos: Short videos explain complex topics in a visually engaging manner, making them accessible to a wide audience. Videos can feature interviews with experts, animations, and personal stories that humanize the impact of AMR.

Live streams and Webinars: Interactive live streams and webinars facilitate real-time discussions and Q&A sessions, allowing viewers to engage directly with experts and gain a deeper understanding of AMR.

Online Resources: Digital platforms provide a space to host and share comprehensive resources, such as interactive websites, e-learning modules, and multimedia toolkits, that educate users about AMR.

Press releases are essential tools for disseminating important updates, milestones, and announcements related to AMR. These concise and factual statements communicate key developments to the media, stakeholders, and the public, ensuring that critical information reaches a wide audience.

- ➤ **Effective press releases include:**
- ➤ Clear Messaging: Press releases deliver concise and jargon-free messages that highlight the significance of the announcement and its relevance to AMR.
- ➤ Timely Dissemination: Press releases are distributed promptly to coincide with events, policy changes, research findings, or awareness campaigns.
- ➤ Contact Information: Contact details for media inquiries ensure that journalists and reporters can access additional information or schedule interviews.

➢ Relevant Quotes: Quotes from experts or key stakeholders add depth and credibility to the press release, conveying the importance of the announcement.

Press releases serve as a bridge between organizations and the media, facilitating accurate reporting and enhancing public understanding of AMR-related developments.

Feature Stories: CDC Solutions

Feature stories are narratives that delve deeper into specific aspects of AMR, providing context, human interest, and insights into the CDC's solutions and initiatives. These stories humanize the impact of AMR by sharing personal experiences, success stories, and the perspectives of healthcare professionals, researchers, and individuals affected by AMR.

Key components of impactful feature stories include:

➢ Personal Narratives: Stories that highlight the experiences of individuals, patients, and healthcare workers shed light on the challenges posed by AMR and the importance of responsible antibiotic use.

- ➤ Success Stories: Narratives about successful interventions, collaborations, or innovations showcase tangible outcomes and inspire hope for addressing AMR.
- ➤ Expert Insights: Expert interviews provide authoritative perspectives that enhance the credibility and depth of the story.
- ➤ Visual Storytelling: Photographs, videos, and multimedia elements enhance the storytelling experience and evoke emotional connections.
- ➤ Feature stories connect readers with the human side of AMR and underscore the CDC's contributions to finding solutions. They offer a platform for showcasing the agency's research, initiatives, and partnerships that are making a positive impact in the fight against AMR.

Communication resources play a pivotal role in advancing the fight against AMR by disseminating accurate information, raising awareness, and inspiring action. From print materials and digital resources to press releases and feature stories, these tools collectively empower individuals and communities to make informed decisions, engage in preventive behaviors, and contribute to the global effort to preserve the effectiveness of antimicrobial agents.

AR Lab Networks: Strengthening Antimicrobial Resistance Surveillance and Research

Antimicrobial resistance (AR) lab networks are collaborative platforms that bring together laboratories, researchers, and public health agencies to enhance surveillance, research, and data sharing related to antimicrobial resistance. These networks play a crucial role in tracking the emergence and spread of resistant microorganisms, understanding resistance mechanisms, and guiding effective interventions to combat AMR. The AR lab networks facilitate a multidisciplinary approach that spans clinical, veterinary, and environmental settings, contributing to a comprehensive understanding of AMR dynamics.

Key features and contributions of AR lab networks include:

> Surveillance and Data Collection: AR lab networks collect and analyze data from diverse sources, including clinical specimens, animal samples, and environmental samples. This

surveillance provides insights into resistance patterns, prevalence, and trends.

➢ Standardized Protocols: Networks establish standardized protocols for laboratory testing, data collection, and reporting, ensuring consistency and comparability of results across different sites.

➢ Capacity Building: AR lab networks provide training, technical assistance, and resources to strengthen the capacity of laboratories in diagnosing and characterizing resistant microorganisms.

➢ Collaboration and Information Sharing: By fostering collaboration between laboratories and public health agencies, AR lab networks facilitate the exchange of information, best practices, and expertise.

➢ Research and Innovation: Networks contribute to research initiatives that explore the genetic basis of resistance, transmission dynamics, and mechanisms of AMR. This research informs the development of new diagnostics and treatment strategies.

➢ Policy and Decision-Making: Data generated by AR lab networks inform policy decisions, guidelines, and interventions aimed at preventing and controlling AMR.

> ➤ Global Health Security: AR lab networks play a crucial role in strengthening global health security by providing early detection and response to emerging AMR threats.

AR lab networks operate at local, national, and international levels, reflecting the interconnected nature of AMR and the need for a coordinated global response. These networks contribute to building a robust evidence base that informs strategies to mitigate the impact of AMR on human and animal health.

AR Isolate Bank: Preserving and Studying Resistant Microorganisms

The AR Isolate Bank serves as a repository for storing and cataloging collections of antimicrobial-resistant microorganisms. This resource plays a pivotal role in advancing research, diagnostics, and treatment development related to antimicrobial resistance. By preserving a diverse array of resistant isolates, the AR Isolate Bank enables researchers and scientists to study the genetic, molecular, and phenotypic characteristics of resistant microorganisms.

Key functions and significance of the AR Isolate Bank include:

> Genomic Analysis: Researchers can conduct genomic sequencing and analysis on stored isolates to uncover genetic mechanisms underlying resistance, trace transmission routes, and identify emerging resistance trends.

> Mechanism Study: The AR Isolate Bank facilitates investigations into the molecular mechanisms by which microorganisms develop resistance to antimicrobial agents.

> Diagnostics Development: Researchers can use isolates to develop and validate new diagnostic tests that rapidly identify resistant strains, enabling timely and targeted treatment.

> Treatment Strategies: Studying resistant isolates informs the development of innovative treatment strategies, including novel antimicrobial agents and combination therapies.

> Surveillance Validation: Isolate banks provide a resource for validating the accuracy and performance of surveillance methods used to track resistance patterns.

> Collaborative Research: The AR Isolate Bank supports collaborative research initiatives that

involve multiple laboratories, institutions, and countries.

- ➢ Education and Training: The bank can be utilized for educational purposes, allowing students, researchers, and healthcare professionals to study and learn about antimicrobial resistance.

The AR Isolate Bank contributes to a deeper understanding of AMR and enhances our ability to respond effectively to this global health threat. By providing a repository of diverse resistant microorganisms, the bank accelerates research and innovation, ultimately aiding in the development of strategies to combat AMR.

Transatlantic Taskforce (TATFAR): Collaborative Efforts in AMR

The Transatlantic Taskforce on Antimicrobial Resistance (TATFAR) is a collaborative initiative that brings together representatives from the United States and European Union (EU) to address the global challenge of antimicrobial resistance. TATFAR seeks to strengthen transatlantic cooperation, share best practices, and develop coordinated strategies to prevent and control AMR.

Key objectives and activities of TATFAR include:

> Policy Coordination: TATFAR facilitates dialogue and collaboration between the U.S. and EU to align policies, regulations, and strategies related to AMR.
> Information Sharing: The task force promotes the exchange of information, data, and experiences in areas such as antimicrobial use, surveillance, and infection prevention and control.
> Best Practice Sharing: TATFAR facilitates the sharing of best practices and lessons learned in tackling AMR, enabling both regions to benefit from each other's experiences.
> Research and Innovation: The task force supports joint research initiatives, innovation, and the development of new tools and interventions to combat AMR.
> One Health Approach: TATFAR recognizes the interconnectedness of human health, animal health, and the environment, and promotes a One Health approach to address AMR.
> Public Engagement: TATFAR engages with stakeholders, including healthcare professionals, researchers, industry, and civil

society, to raise awareness and mobilize action against AMR.

➤ Policy Recommendations: The task force develops policy recommendations and action plans that guide the U.S. and EU in their efforts to address AMR.

TATFAR exemplifies the importance of international collaboration in the fight against AMR. By leveraging the expertise, resources, and experiences of both the U.S. and EU, TATFAR contributes to a unified and coordinated global response to the growing threat of antimicrobial resistance. Through joint efforts, TATFAR aims to safeguard the efficacy of antimicrobial agents and protect public health on both sides of the Atlantic.

Conclusion

In the face of a rapidly escalating global health crisis, the initiatives outlined – the AR Lab Networks, the AR Isolate Bank, and the Transatlantic Taskforce (TATFAR) – stand as pillars of strength and innovation in the battle against antimicrobial resistance (AMR). These initiatives collectively exemplify the power of collaboration, data-driven research, and international cooperation in addressing one of the most pressing challenges of our time.

The AR Lab Networks epitomize the essence of a comprehensive, multidisciplinary approach. By uniting laboratories, researchers, and public health agencies across various sectors, these networks weave a tapestry of data that unveils the intricate patterns of AMR. Through standardized protocols, capacity-building efforts, and robust collaboration, these networks provide the critical surveillance needed to track the evolution and spread of resistant microorganisms. They not only enhance our understanding of AMR dynamics but also underpin evidence-based interventions that can shape policies, guide clinical practices, and secure the foundations of global health security.

The AR Isolate Bank serves as an invaluable repository of hope and knowledge. In its genetic sequences, scientists unearth the secrets of resistance mechanisms, unlocking insights that may shape the development of novel diagnostics, innovative treatments, and sustainable solutions. This living library of resistance accelerates research, offering an arsenal of resources to combat the threat of antimicrobial resistance. As researchers dissect the genetic blueprints of resistance, the AR Isolate Bank stands as a beacon of discovery, poised to illuminate the path toward new therapeutic horizons.

The Transatlantic Taskforce (TATFAR) stands as a testament to the power of international collaboration in the face of a global health threat. Bridging the Atlantic, this partnership between the United States and the European Union epitomizes unity and shared responsibility. Through dialogue, policy coordination, and the exchange of best practices, TATFAR forges a transatlantic alliance that confronts AMR head-on. As the world grapples with the complexity of AMR, TATFAR stands as a symbol of the potential when nations transcend borders and work together toward a common goal.

In this intensive exploration of initiatives against AMR, a profound narrative emerges – a narrative of resilience, innovation, and unwavering determination. The AR Lab Networks, the AR Isolate Bank, and TATFAR encapsulate the essence of a united response to a formidable global challenge. They represent the embodiment of science, collaboration, and international solidarity, showing that in the pursuit of a world without the looming shadow of AMR, the collective efforts of nations, communities, and individuals hold the key to a brighter, healthier future. As we move forward, these initiatives stand as beacons of hope, guiding us through the complex labyrinth of AMR toward a horizon where antimicrobial agents remain effective, human health is safeguarded, and the resounding call for action becomes an indomitable force for change.

References

Abbate, E., Vescovo, M., Natiello, M., Cufré, M., García, A., Montaner, P. G., et al. (2012). Successful alternative treatment of extensively drug-resistant tuberculosis in Argentina with a combination of linezolid, moxifloxacin and thioridazine. J. Antimicrobial. Chemother.

Adams, K. N., Szumowski, J. D., Ramakrishnan, L. (2014). Verapamil, and its metabolite norverapamil, inhibit macrophage-induced, bacterial efflux pump-mediated tolerance to multiple anti-tubercular drugs. J. Infect. Dis. 210, 456–466. doi: 10.1093/infdis/jiu095

Adams, K. N., Takaki, K., Connolly, L. E., Wiedenhoft, H., Winglee, K., Humbert, O., et al. (2011). Drug tolerance in replicating mycobacteria mediated by a macrophage-induced efflux mechanism.

Adams, K. N., Verma, A. K., Gopalaswamy, R., Adikesavalu, H., Singhal, D. K., Tripathy, S., et al. (2019). Diverse clinical isolates of Mycobacterium tuberculosis develop macrophage-induced rifampin tolerance. J. Infect.

Amaral, L., Kristiansen, J. E., Viveiros, M., Atouguia, J. (2001). Activity of phenothiazines against antibiotic-resistant Mycobacterium tuberculosis: a review supporting further studies that may elucidate the potential use of thioridazine as anti-tuberculosis therapy. J. Antimicrob. Chemother.

Amaral, L., Viveiros, M. (2017). Thioridazine: A non-antibiotic drug highly effective, in combination with first line anti-tuberculosis drugs, against any form of antibiotic resistance of Mycobacterium tuberculosis due to its multi-mechanisms of action. Antibiotics 6. doi: 10.3390/antibiotics6010003

Antonelli, A., D'Andrea, M. M., Brenciani, A., Galeotti, C. L., Morroni, G., Pollini, S., et al. (2018). Characterization of poxtA, a novel phenicol-oxazolidinone-tetracycline resistance gene from an MRSA of clinical origin. J. Antimicrobial. Chemother.

Antonova-Koch, Y., Meister, S., Abraham, M., Luth, M. R., Ottilie, S., Lukens, A. K., et al. (2018). Open-source discovery of chemical leads for next-generation chemoprotective antimalarials. Science 1979) 362, 1129. doi: 10.1126/science.aat9446

Ates, L. S., Ummels, R., Commandeur, S., van de Weerd, R., van der Weerd, R., Sparrius, M., et al. (2015). Essential role of the ESX-5 secretion system in outer membrane permeability of pathogenic mycobacteria.

Balaban, N. Q., Helaine, S., Lewis, K., Ackermann, M., Aldridge, B., Andersson, D. I., et al. (2019). Definitions and guidelines for research on antibiotic persistence.

Banerjee, A., Dubnau, E., Quemard, A., Balasubramanian, V., Um, K. S., Wilson, T., et al. (1994). inhA, a gene encoding a target for isoniazid and ethionamide in Mycobacterium tuberculosis.

Bateson, A., Ortiz Canseco, J., McHugh, T. D., Witney, A. A., Feuerriegel, S., Merker, M., et al. (2022). Ancient and recent differences in the intrinsic susceptibility of Mycobacterium tuberculosis complex to pretomanid. J. Antimicrob. Chemother.

Batt, S. M., Minnikin, D. E., Besra, G. S. (2020). The thick waxy coat of mycobacteria, a protective layer against antibiotics and the host's immune system. Biochem. J

Boritsch, E. C., Khanna, V., Pawlik, A., Honoré, N., Navas, V. H., Ma, L., et al. (2016). Key experimental evidence of chromosomal DNA transfer among selected tuberculosis-causing mycobacteria. Proc.

Borrell, S., Trauner, A., Brites, D., Rigouts, L., Loiseau, C., Coscolla, M., et al. (2019). Reference set of Mycobacterium tuberculosis clinical strains: A tool for research and product development.

Bosch, B., DeJesus, M. A., Poulton, N. C., Zhang, W., Engelhart, C. A., Zaveri, A., et al. (2021). Genome-wide gene expression tuning reveals diverse vulnerabilities of M. tuberculosis.

Boyer, E., Dessolin, J., Lustig, M., Decossas, M., Phan, G., Cece, Q., et al. (2022). Molecular determinants for OMF selectivity in tripartite RND multidrug efflux systems. Antibiot. (Basel). 11

Braibant, M., Gilot, P., Content, J. (2000). The ATP binding cassette (ABC) transport systems of Mycobacterium tuberculosis.

Brauner, A., Fridman, O., Gefen, O., Balaban, N. Q. (2016). Distinguishing between resistance, tolerance and persistence to antibiotic treatment.

Briffotaux, J., Huang, W., Wang, X., Gicquel, B. (2017). MmpS5/MmpL5 as an efflux pump in Mycobacterium species. Tuberculosis

Brown, J. C. S., Nelson, J., Vandersluis, B., Deshpande, R., Butts, A., Kagan, S., et al. (2014). Unraveling the biology of a fungal meningitis pathogen using chemical genetics.

Burian, J., Yim, G., Hsing, M., Axerio-Cilies, P., Cherkasov, A., Spiegelman, G. B., et al. (2013). The mycobacterial antibiotic resistance determinant WhiB7 acts as a transcriptional activator by binding the primary sigma factor SigA (RpoV). Nucleic Acids Res. 41, 10062–10076. doi: 10.1093/nar/gkt751

Cacace, E., Kritikos, G., Typas, A. (2017). Chemical genetics in drug discovery. Curr. Opin. Syst.

Campbell, E. A., Korzheva, N., Mustaev, A., Murakami, K., Nair, S., Goldfarb, A., et al. (2001). Structural mechanism for rifampicin inhibition of bacterial RNA polymerase.

Capobianco, J. O., Cao, Z., Shortridge, V. D., Ma, Z., Flamm, R. K., Zhong, P. (2000). Studies of the novel ketolide ABT-773: Transport, binding to ribosomes, and inhibition of protein synthesis in Streptococcus pneumoniae. Antimicrob. Agents Chemother

Carey, A. F., Rock, J. M., Krieger, I., Chase, M. R., Fernandez-Suarez, M., Gagneux, S., et al. (2018). TnSeq of Mycobacterium tuberculosis clinical isolates reveals strain-specific antibiotic liabilities.

Chen, C., Gardete, S., Jansen, R. S., Shetty, A., Dick, T., Rhee, K. Y., et al. (2018). Verapamil targets membrane energetics in Mycobacterium tuberculosis. Antimicrob. Agents Chemother

Choudhary, E., Thakur, P., Pareek, M., Agarwal, N. (2015). Gene silencing by CRISPR interference in mycobacteria.

Coe, K. A., Lee, W., Stone, M. C., Komazin-Meredith, G., Meredith, T. C., Grad, Y. H., et al. (2019). Multi-strain tn-seq reveals common daptomycin resistance determinants in Staphylococcus aureus

Coelho, T., Machado, D., Couto, I., Maschmann, R., Ramos, D., von Groll, A., et al. (2015). Enhancement of antibiotic activity by efflux inhibitors against multidrug resistant Mycobacterium tuberculosis clinical isolates from Brazil. Front. Microbiol.

Cokol, M., Kuru, N., Bicak, E., Larkins-Ford, J., Aldridge, B. B. (2017). Efficient measurement and factorization of high-order drug interactions in Mycobacterium tuberculosis. Sci. Adv. 3, e170188. doi: 10.1126/sciadv.1701881